BALANCE

EXERCISES

FOR WOMEN OVER 50

The comprehensive 30 days challenge to improve strength, posture and flexibility

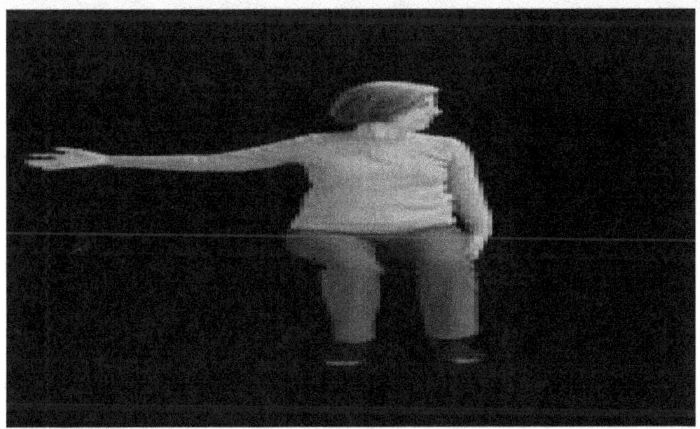

JAMES CORDERO–

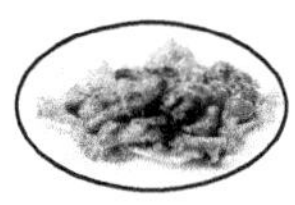 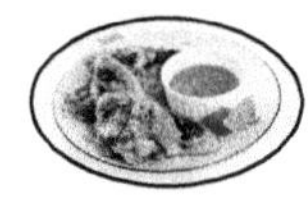 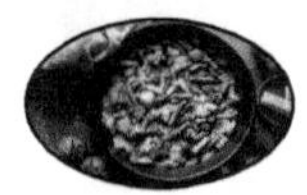

Copyright Page

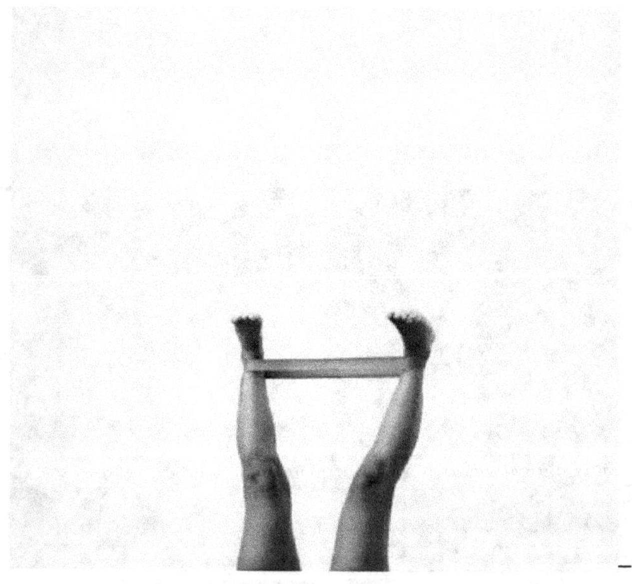

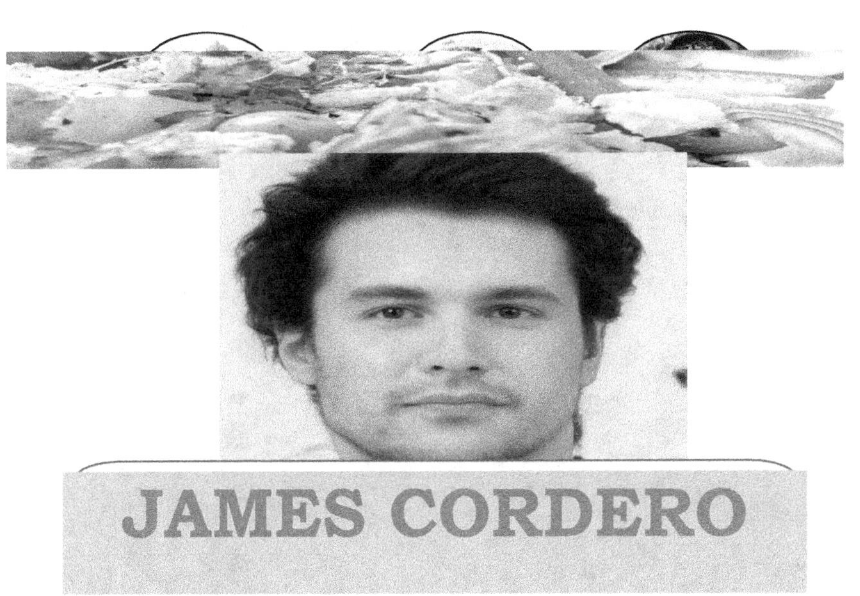

JAMES CORDERO

James Cordero is a devoted yoga and Pilate's instructor, deeply committed to guiding individuals on a transformative journey of self-discovery, where the intricate connection between body and mind takes center stage. With a wealth of expertise in both disciplines, James brings a fresh perspective to traditional Pilate's routines by seamlessly incorporating the use of the wall, making these practices accessible to individuals of all ages and experience levels.

In his role as an instructor, James goes beyond the physical aspects of fitness, emphasizing the holistic nature of well-being. His teachings inspire a profound exploration of the harmonious relationship between body, mind, and spirit,

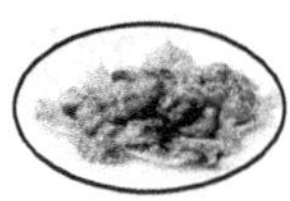 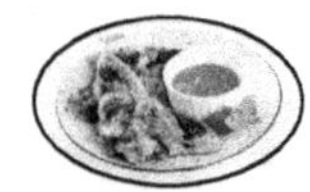 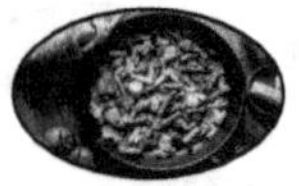

fostering a sense of equilibrium that extends far beyond the confines of her classes.

Outside the studio, James seeks solace in the embrace of nature, finding inspiration in the pages of literature, and cherishing moments shared with loved ones. His dedication to empowering individuals on their holistic wellness journey serves as a testament to James's unwavering commitment as a yoga and Pilates practitioner.

Known for his creative and professional approach, James Cordero is not just an instructor; he is a guide, mentor, and advocate for a balanced and fulfilling life, embodying the essence of holistic well-being in every aspect of her work.

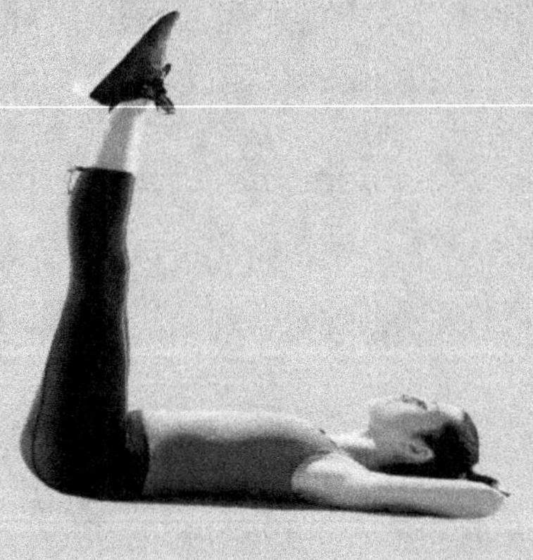

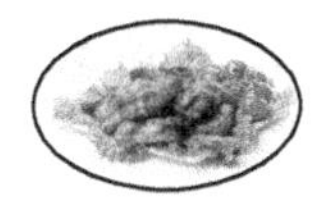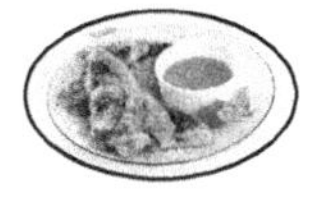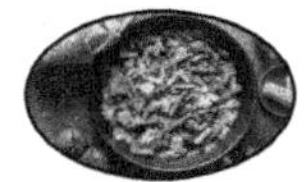

TABLE OF CONTENT

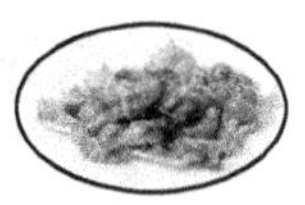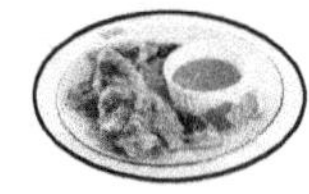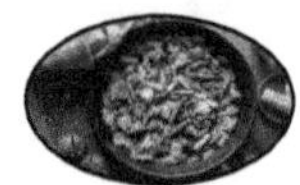

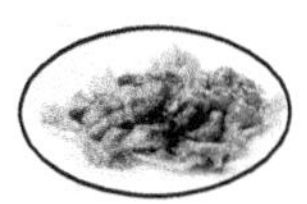
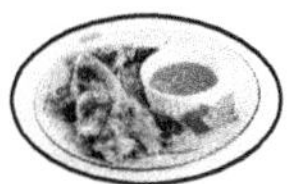
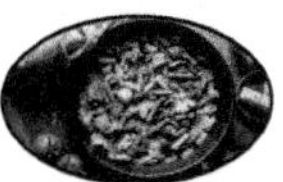
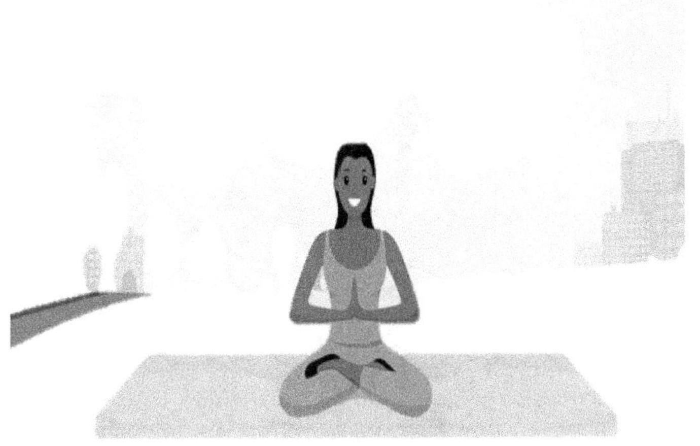
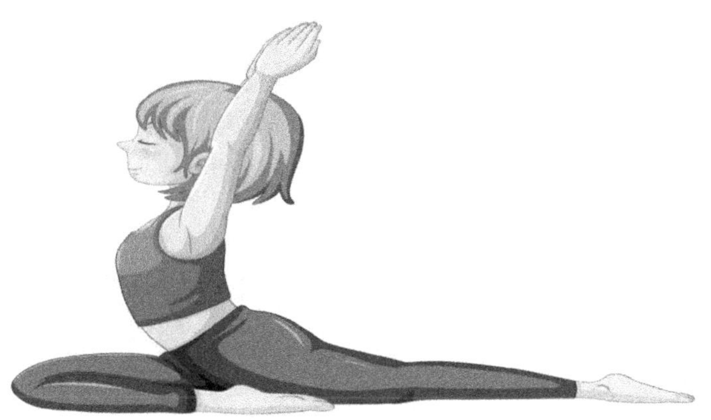

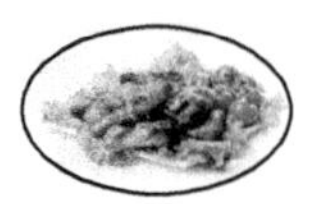 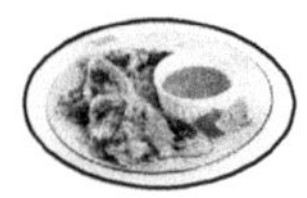 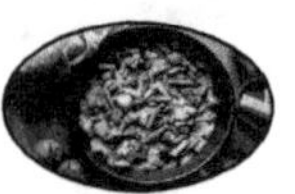

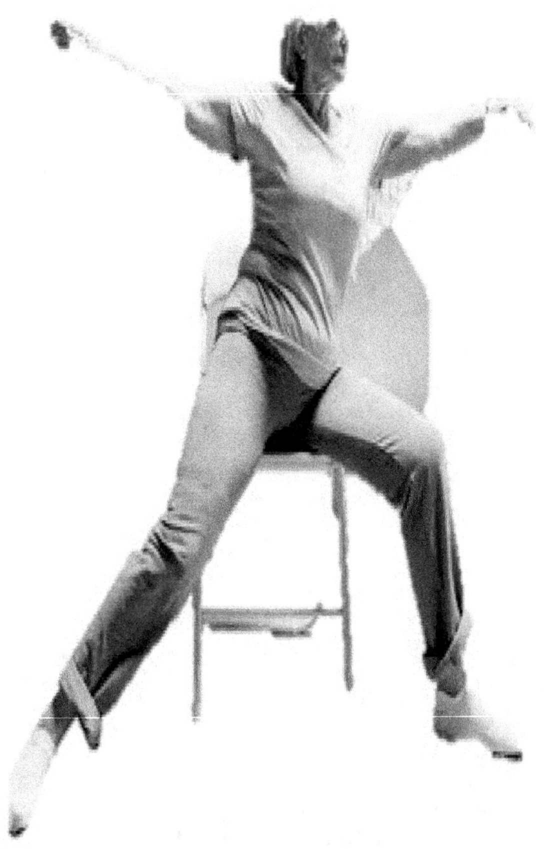

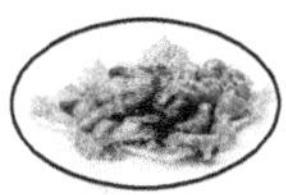
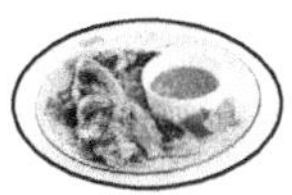
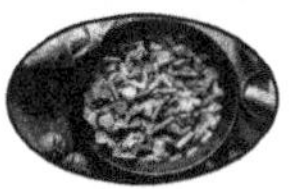

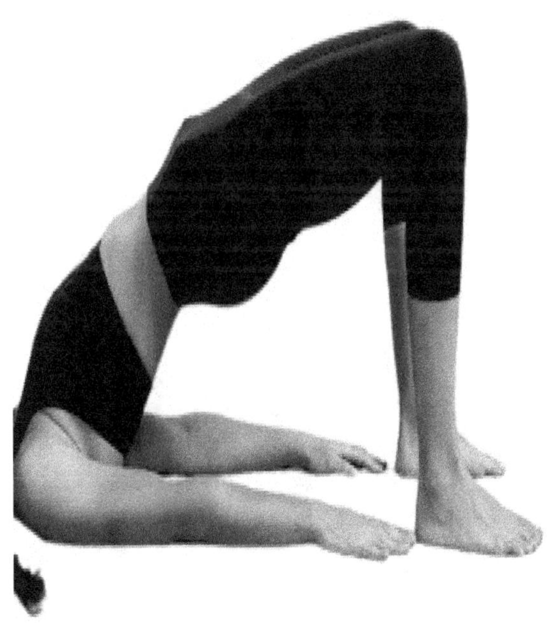

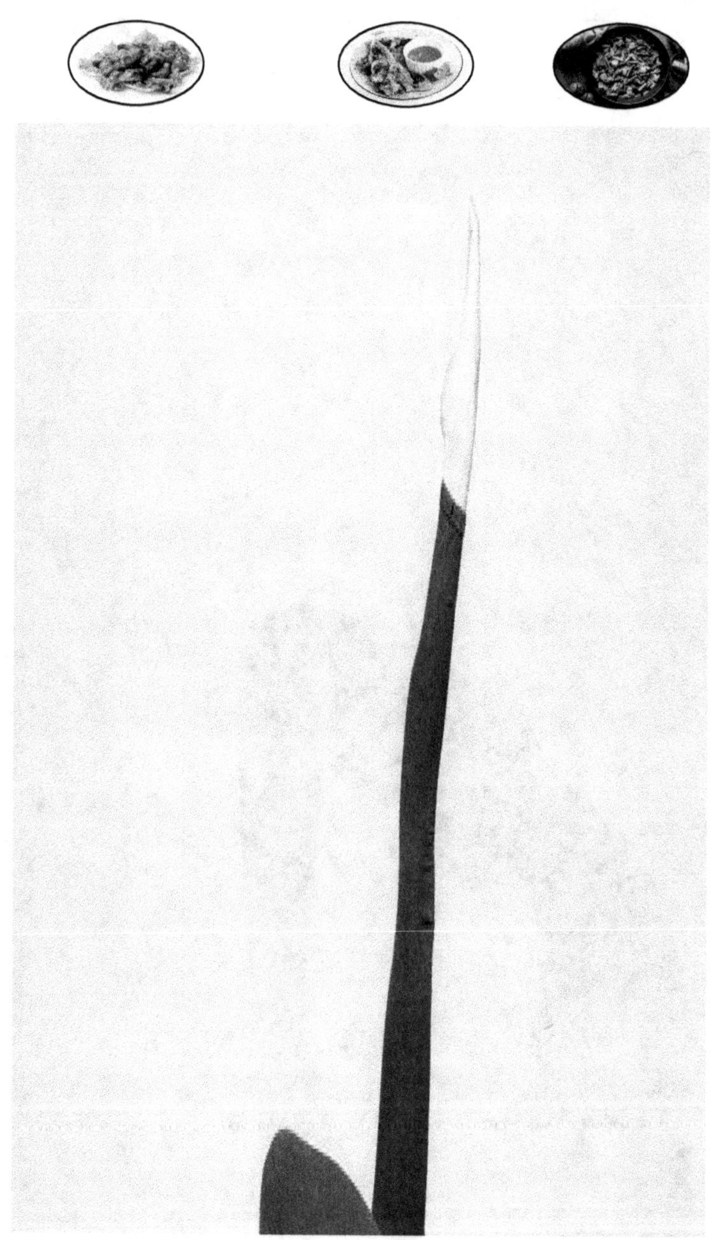

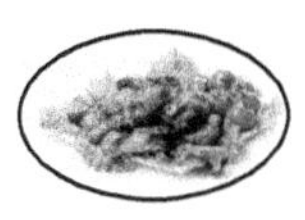 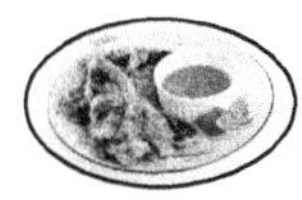 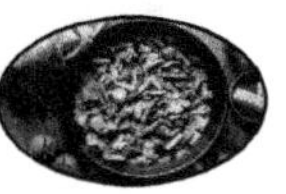

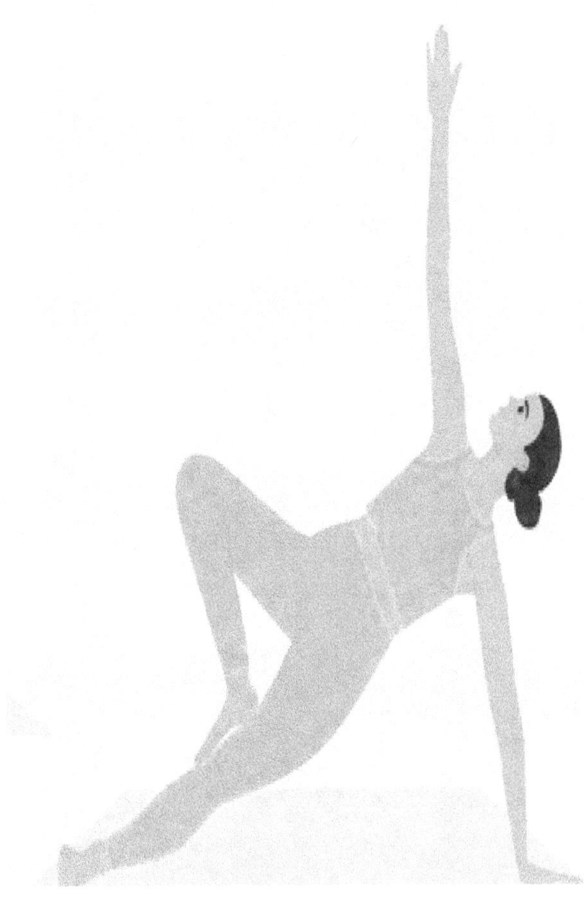

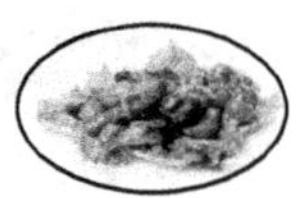 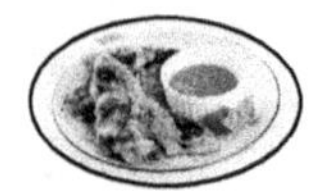 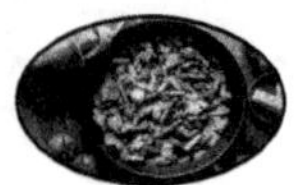

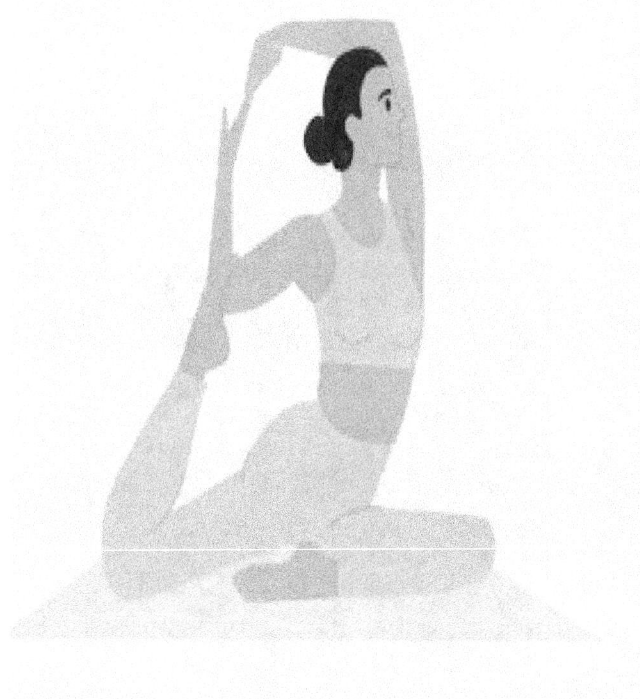

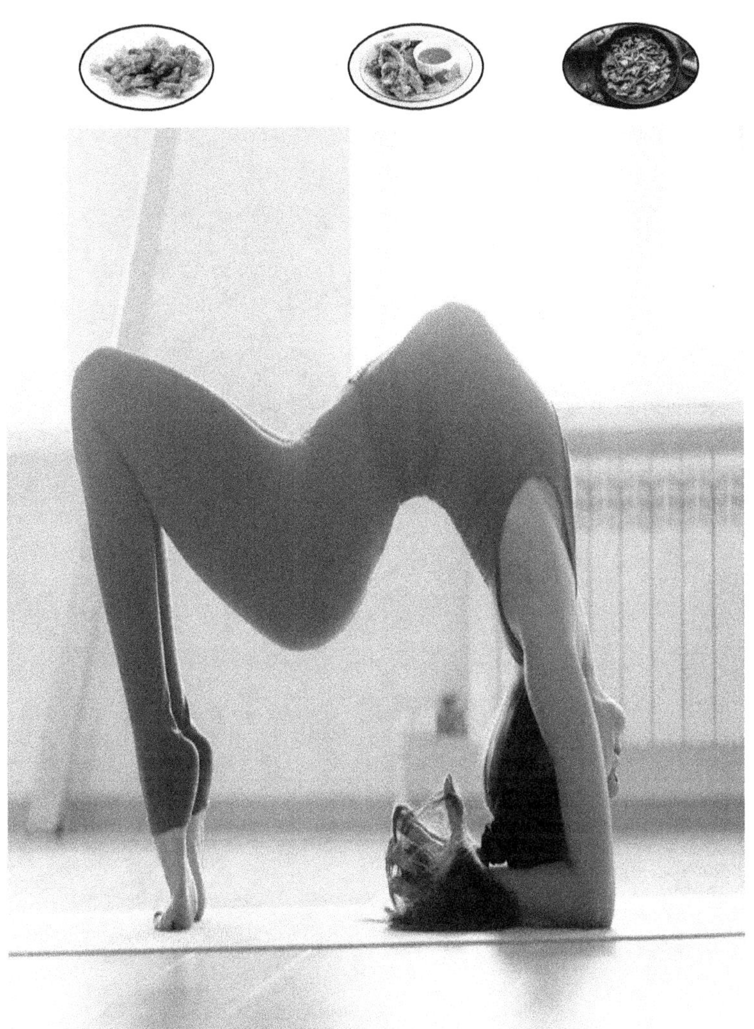

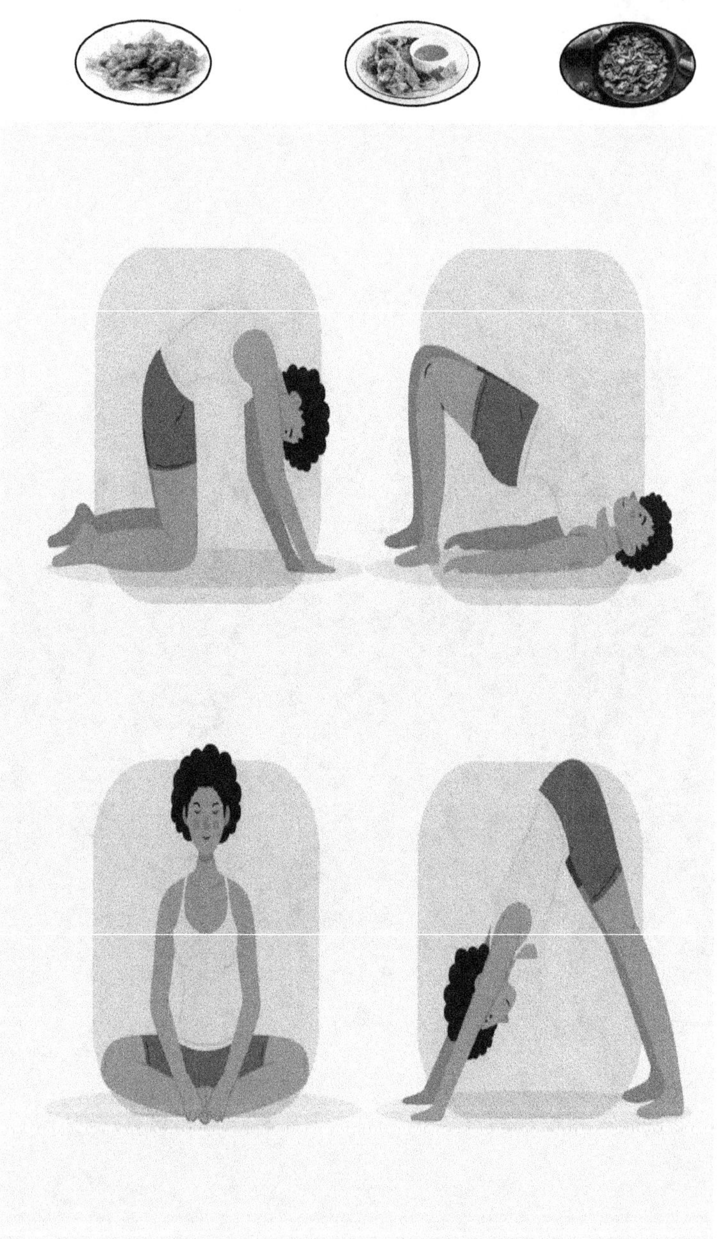

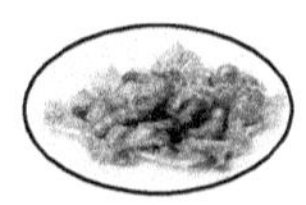 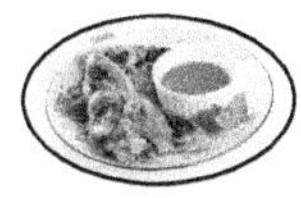 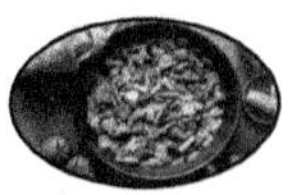

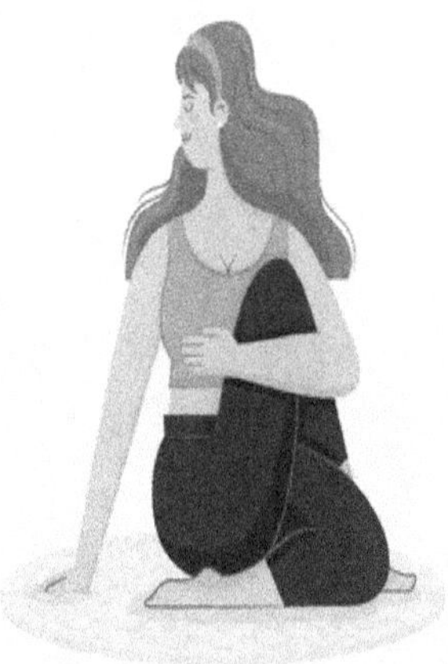 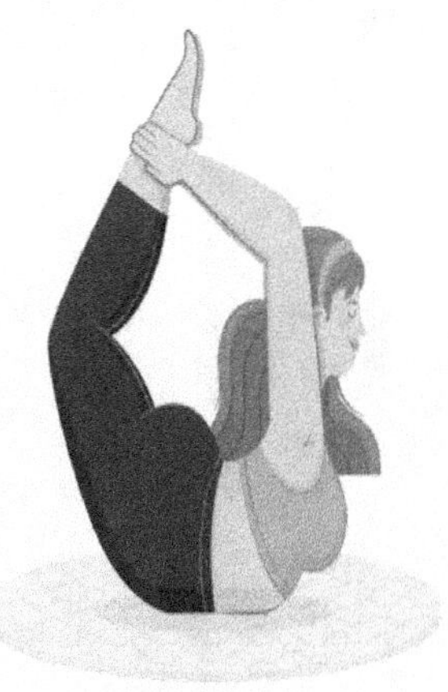

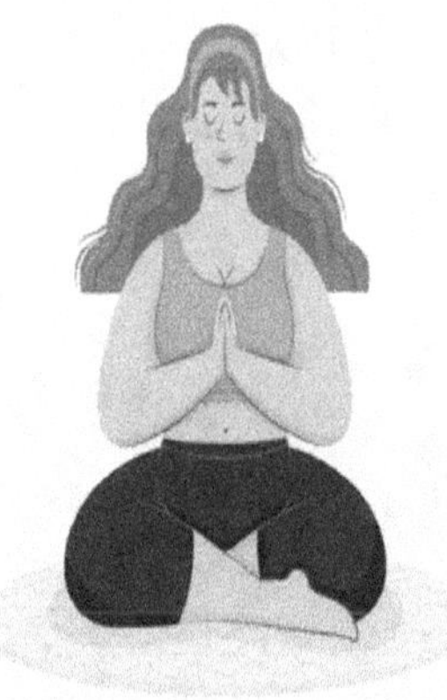 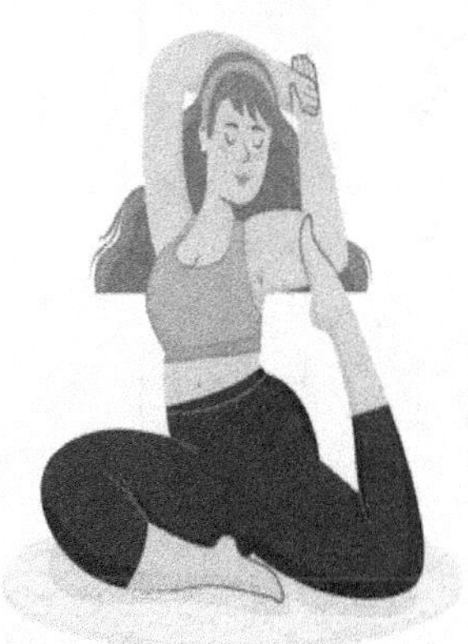

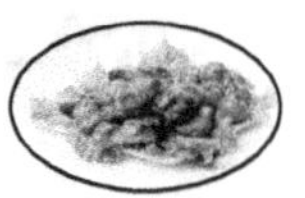 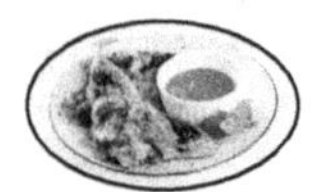 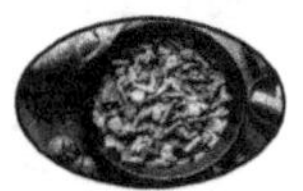

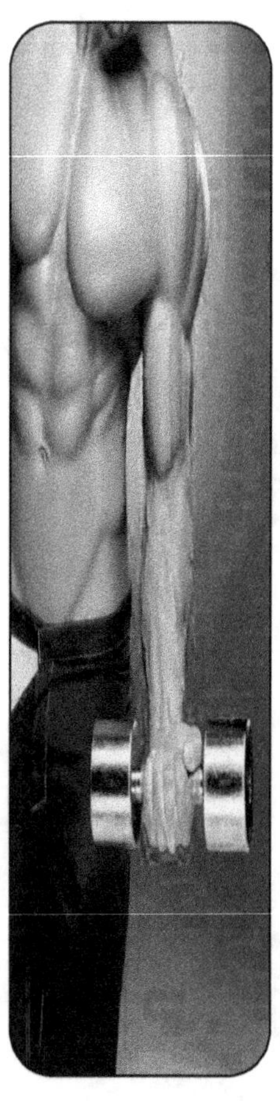 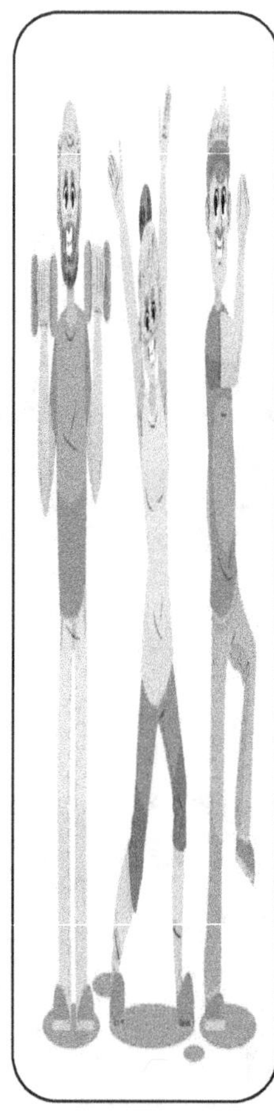 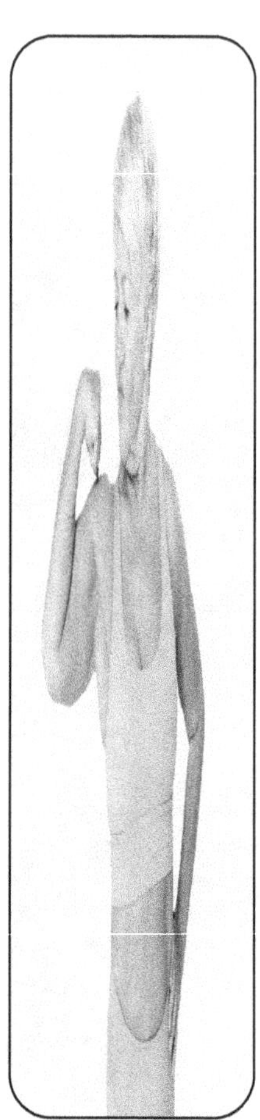

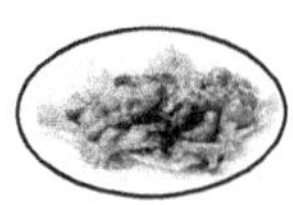 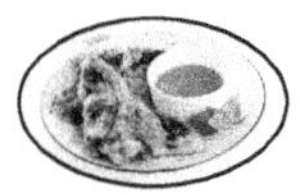 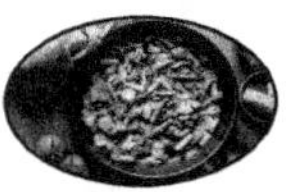

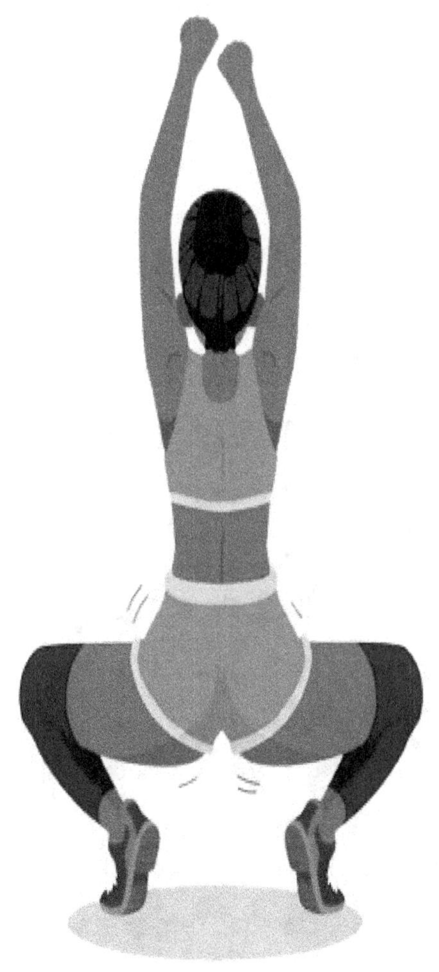

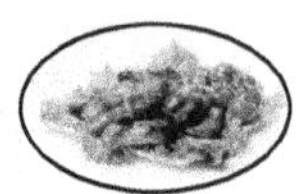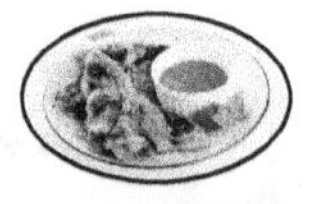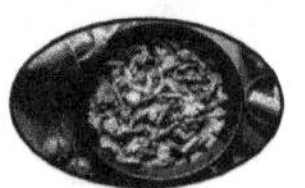

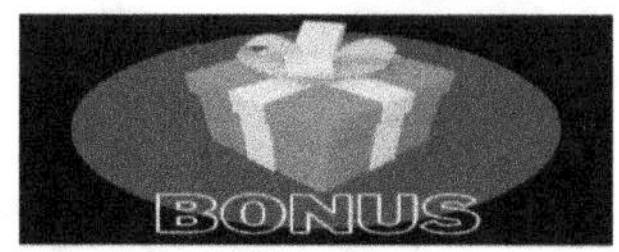

SCAN THE QR CODE TO GET YOUR FREE HOME MADE GREEN SMOOTHIE RECIPE BOOK

BONUS 1

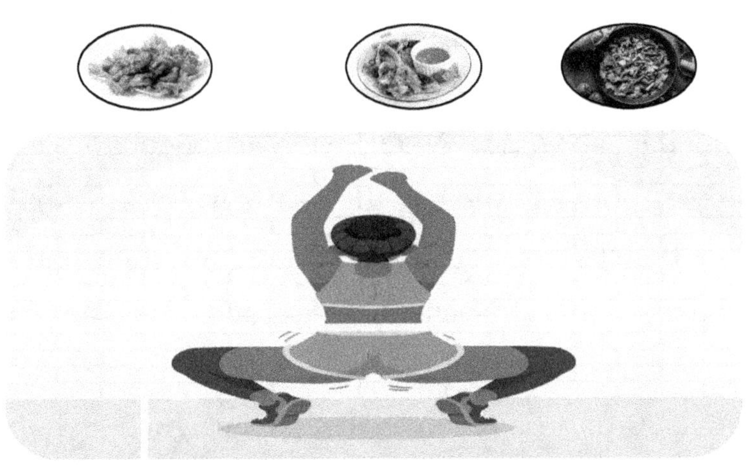

INTRODUCTION–

In the quaint town of Harmony Springs, where time seemed to slow down, three remarkable women in their 50s discovered a secret to rejuvenating their lives. The whispers of an unconventional 30-day challenge echoed through the community, promising not just physical transformation but a revival of spirit. This challenge, a tapestry woven with 40 distinct balance exercises, became a lifeline for Amelia, Grace, and Olivia, three friends whose journeys were about to intersect in the most unexpected way.–

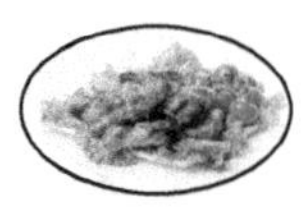 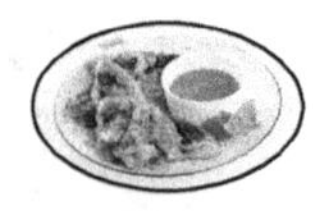 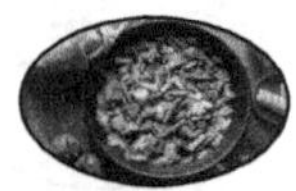

Amelia, a vibrant soul with a penchant for adventure, felt the weight of years settling into her bones. Her days of climbing mountains and chasing sunsets seemed distant memories as the relentless march of time took its toll. The prospect of a 30-day balance challenge intrigued her, a glimmer of hope in the routine of her life. Little did she know that it would be the catalyst for a profound metamorphosis.

Grace, a woman of elegance and grace, found herself caught in the snares of a sedentary lifestyle. The once-fluid movements that defined her dance with life were gradually replaced by the stiffness of inactivity. Longing for the days when her posture exuded confidence, Grace eagerly embraced the challenge, seeking not just physical resilience but a rekindling of the poise that had waltzed away over the years.–

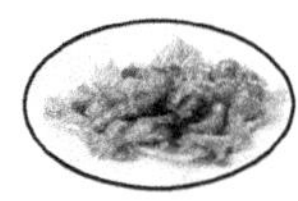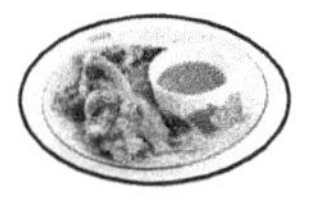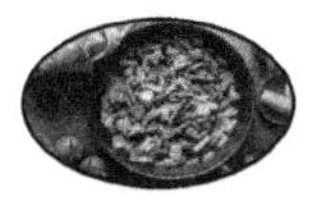

Olivia, a quiet force with a heart full of dreams, faced the silent battles of aging. The mirror reflected changes that whispered doubts, and her strength, both physical and emotional, seemed to wane. The 30-day challenge presented itself as a beacon of strength, a chance to rewrite the narrative and carve a path toward resilience.

As the three women embarked on this shared journey, their lives intertwined in the rhythm of daily exercises. Wall squats, tree poses, and balancing bird poses became not just movements but verses in a symphony of rejuvenation. Each day brought new challenges, and with them, newfound strengths.

Amelia, the adventurer, felt her muscles awaken from a deep slumber. The wall squats that once seemed daunting became a testament to her tenacity. With each controlled descent, she not only strengthened her quads but unearthed –

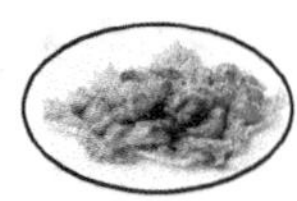 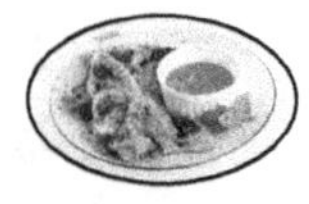 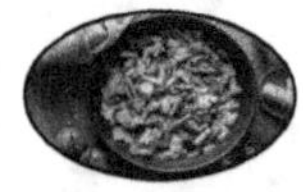

a reservoir of determination that had long laid dormant. The benefits of improved strength resonated not only in her physicality but in the renewed twinkle in her eyes.

For Grace, the dance of the 30-day challenge was a ballet of rediscovery. The fluidity of the tree pose, the elegance of the figure 4 stretch – each movement carried her back to the ballrooms of her youth. With each day, her posture transformed, shedding the cloak of stiffness to reveal the grace that had never truly left her. Her newfound poise radiated not only in her body but in the confidence that permeated her every step.

As for Olivia, the wall leg lifts became a metaphor for lifting the burdens that had settled on her shoulders. The rhythmic motion brought not only strength to her hip flexors but also a sense of liberation. With each lift, she shed the weight of doubt, and in the quiet moments of balance, she found the resilience to face the challenges that life presented.

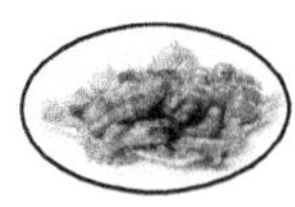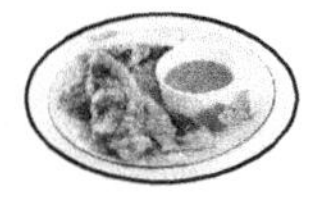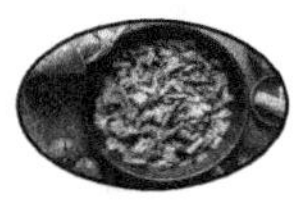

In Harmony Springs, the winds of change whispered through the lives of Amelia, Grace, and Olivia. The 30-day challenge, a seemingly simple tapestry of exercises, wove a narrative of strength, posture, and balance. Their stories, though unique, converged in a shared realization – that age was not a barrier but a canvas waiting to be painted with the vibrant hues of rejuvenation. The challenge became a testament to the transformative power of movement, an ode to the resilience that resides within, waiting to be awakened.

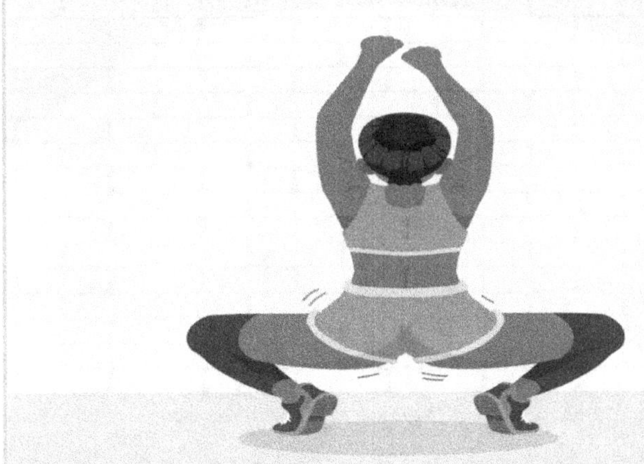

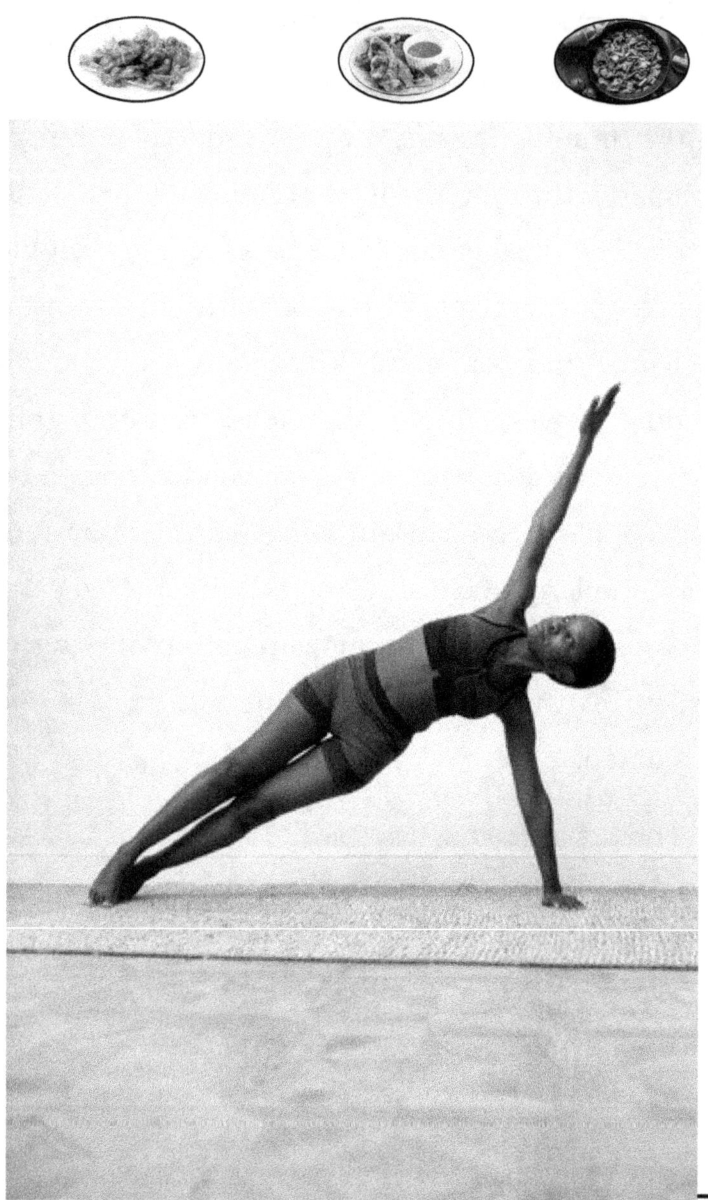

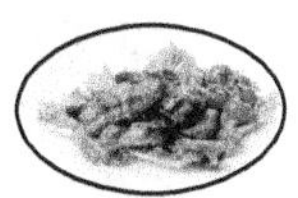 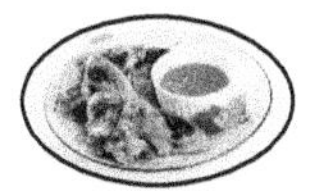 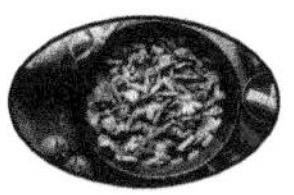

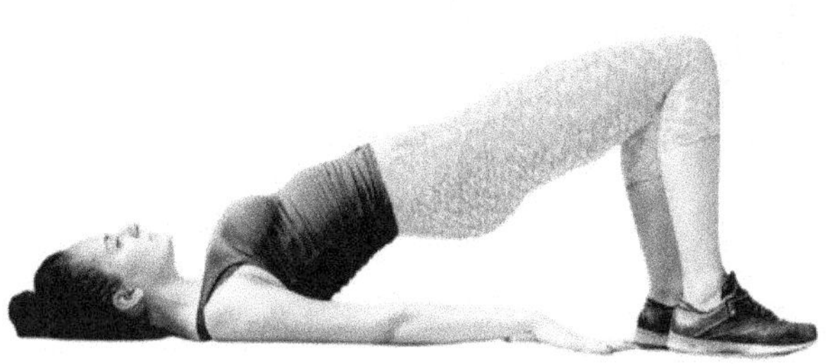

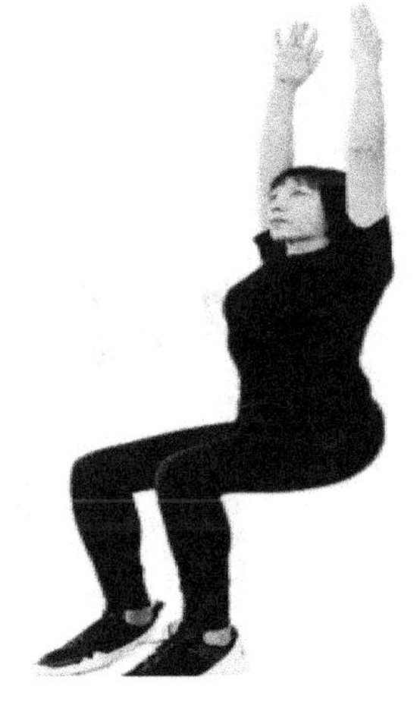

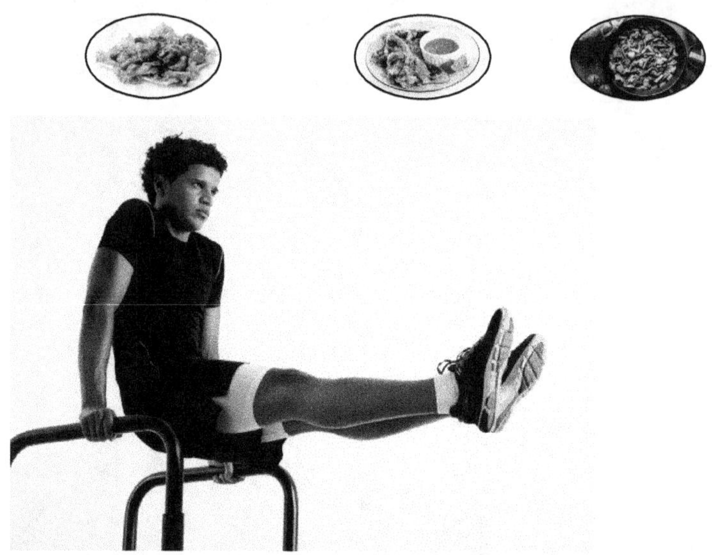

Wall Side Plank

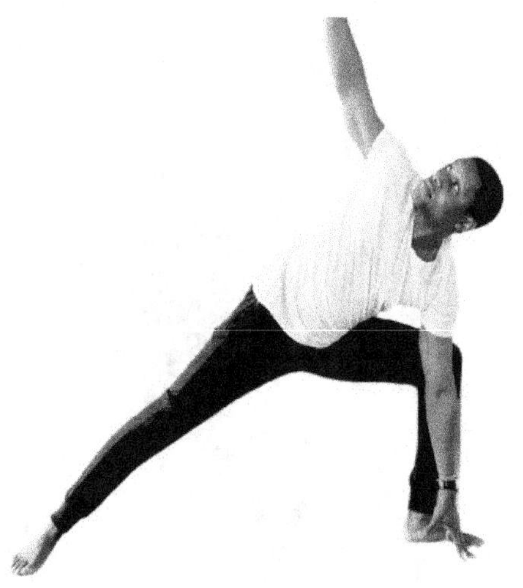

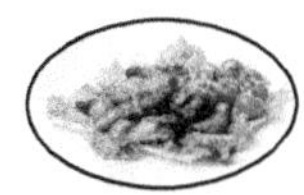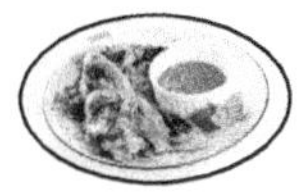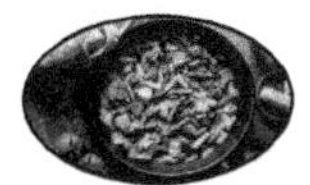

1. Wall Squats

Benefits:

- Strengthens quadriceps and glutes

- Improves overall lower body strength and stability

Steps:

1. Stand with your back against the wall and feet hip-width apart.

2. Slide down the wall, bending your knees, until thighs are parallel to the ground.

3. Hold for 15-30 seconds, then stand back up.

4. Repeat 10-15 times.

Remember:

- Keep your back straight against the wall.

- Don't let your knees go past your toes.

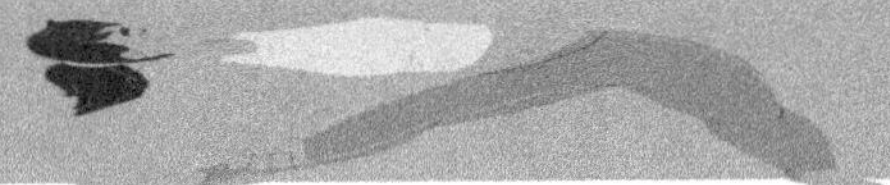

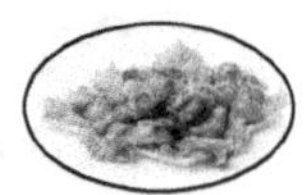 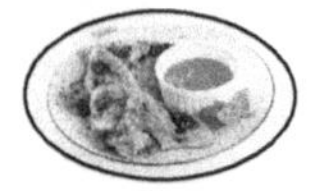 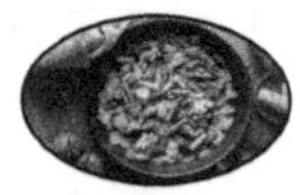

2. Wall Calf Raises

Benefits:

- Strengthens calf muscles

- Enhances ankle stability

Steps:

1. Stand facing the wall with hands resting on it.

2. Lift your heels off the ground, rising onto your toes.

3. Hold for a moment, then lower heels back down.

4. Repeat 15-20 times.

Remember:

- Maintain a straight line from head to heels.

- Control the movement throughout.–

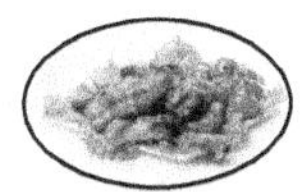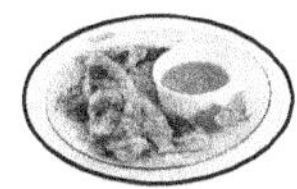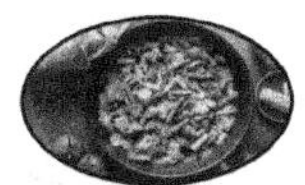

3. Wall Plank

Benefits:

- Strengthens core muscles

- Improves overall body stability

Steps:

1. Spread your hands shoulder-width apart on the wall.

2. Take a step backward until your torso is straight.

3. Hold while using your core for 20 to 30 seconds.

Repeat three to five times.

Keep in mind to: • Maintain a plank posture.

• Keep your hips from sagging.

4. Wall Leg Lifts

Benefits:

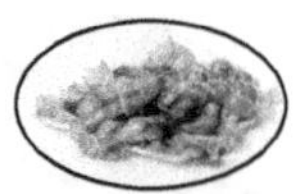 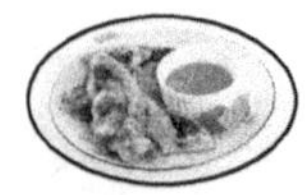 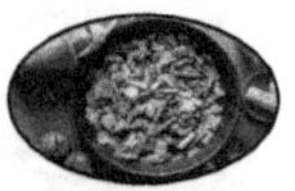

- Targets the hip flexors and lower abdominal muscles

- Improves hip mobility

Steps:

1. Stand facing the wall with hands resting on it.

2. Elevate a single leg straight ahead of you.

3. Hold for 10-15 seconds, then lower the leg.

4. Repeat on the other leg.

Remember:

- • Maintain an active core.

- Regulate the leg's motion.

5. Wall Marching

Benefits:

- Activates core muscles

- Enhances balance and coordination–

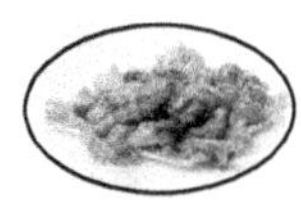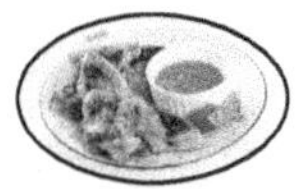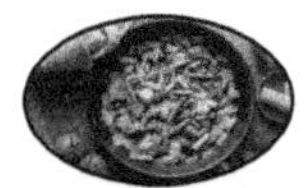

Steps:

1. Stand facing the wall with hands on it.

2. Lift one knee toward your chest, then switch legs.

3. Continue alternating legs for 20-30 seconds.

Remember:

- Maintain a steady pace.

- Keep your back straight.

6. Wall Side Leg Lifts

Benefits:

- Targets outer thighs and hip abductors

- Improves hip and pelvic stability

Steps:

1. Stand sideways to the wall with one hand on it for support.

2. Lift one leg to the side, then lower it.–

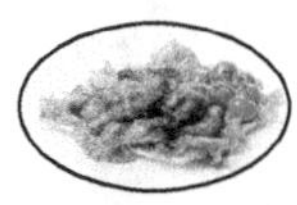 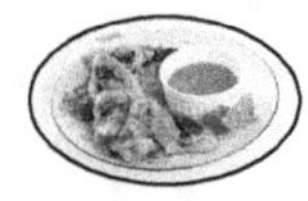 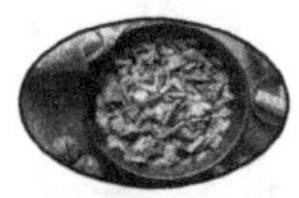

3. Repeat on each side for 15-20 reps.

Remember:

- Keep your core engaged.

- Control the leg movement.

7. Wall Chest Press

Benefits:

- Strengthens chest and arm muscles

- Improves upper body strength

Steps:

1. Stand facing the wall with arms extended.

2. Bend your elbows, bringing your chest toward the wall.

3. Push back to the starting position.

4. Repeat 12-15 times.–

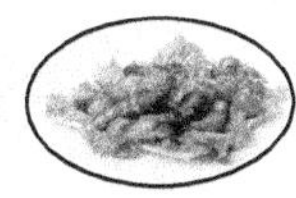 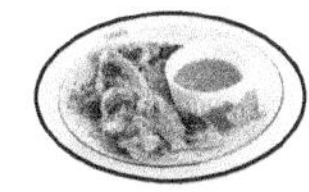 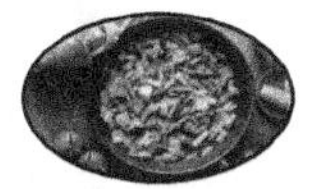

Remember:

- Keep your body in a straight line.

- Control the movement with your chest muscles.

8. Wall Tricep Dips

Benefits:

• Focuses on the upper back and triceps muscles

• Enhances tone and arm strength Steps:

steps

Keeping your back to the wall, place your hands shoulder-width apart on it.

2. Bend your elbows to lower your body.

3. Elevate yourself back to the beginning position.

Ten to twelve times, repeat.

—

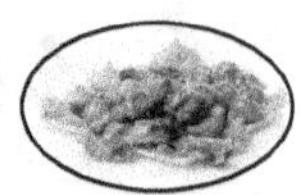 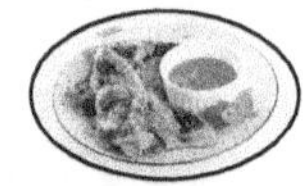 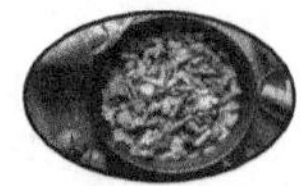

Remember:

- Keep your back close to the wall.

- Control the movement with your triceps.

9. Wall Shoulder Taps

Benefits:

- Activates core muscles

- Improves shoulder stability

Steps:

1. Get into a wall plank position.

2. Lift one hand to tap the opposite shoulder.

3. Alternate sides for 20-30 seconds.

Remember:

- Keep your hips stable.

- Control the tapping motion.–

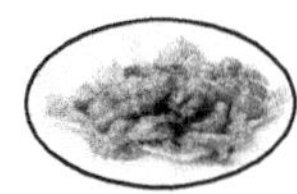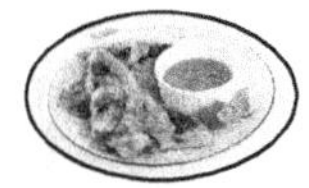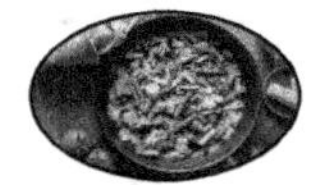

10. Wall Back Extensions

Benefits:

- Targets lower back muscles

- Improves spinal flexibility

Steps:

1. Stand facing the wall with hands on it.

2. Arch your back, reaching your chest towards the wall.

3. Hold for 15-20 seconds, then return to the starting position.

Remember:

- Engage your core.

- Avoid overextending your back.

11. Wall Toe Taps

Benefits:–

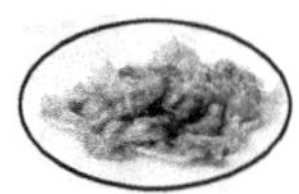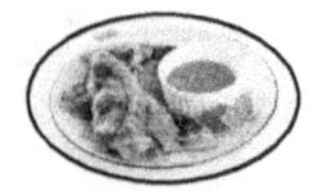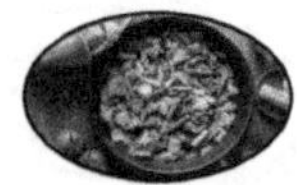

- Engages core muscles

- Enhances lower abdominal strength

Steps:

1. Lie on your back with legs extended up the wall.

2. Lower one leg down toward the floor.

3. Tap the wall with your toes, then lift the leg back up.

4. Repeat on the other leg.

Remember:

- Keep your lower back pressed into the floor.

- Control the movement with your core.

12. Wall Bicycle Crunches

Benefits:

- Targets obliques and abdominal muscles

- Improves overall core strength–

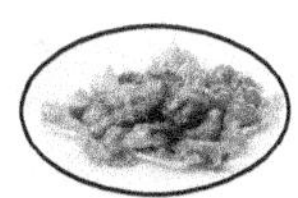 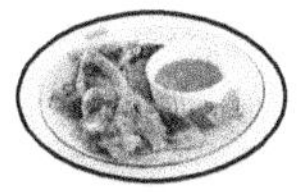 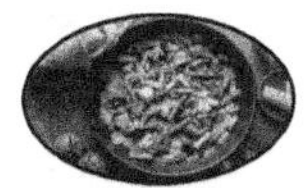

Steps:

1. Lie on your back with legs up the wall.

2. Bring one knee towards your chest while twisting your torso.

3. Extend the opposite leg straight out.

4. Repeat on the other side.

Remember:

- Engage your core throughout.

- Maintain a controlled, twisting motion.

13. Wall Hip Bridges

Benefits:

- Activates glutes and hamstrings

- Improves hip stability and strength

Steps:

1. Lie on your back with feet on the wall, hip-width apart.–

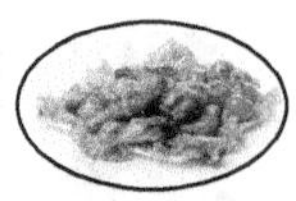 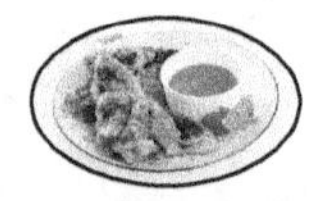 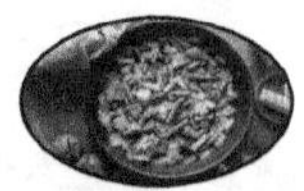

2. Lift your hips towards the ceiling.

3. Hold for 15-20 seconds, then lower back down.

Remember:

- Squeeze your glutes at the top.

- Keep your back straight.

14. Wall Side Plank

Benefits:

- Strengthens core and oblique muscles

- Improves lateral stability

Steps:

1. Lie on your side with feet against the wall.

2. Lift your hips, creating a straight line from head to heels.

3. Hold for 20-30 seconds on each side.–

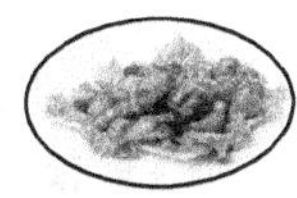 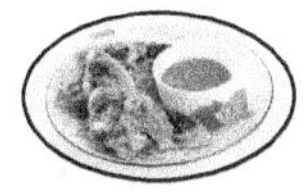 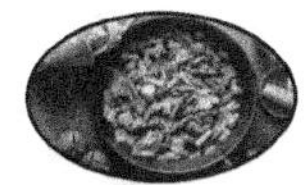

Remember:

- Keep your body in a straight line.

- Engage your obliques.

15. Wall Chest Squeeze

Benefits:

- Targets chest muscles and improves posture

- Enhances shoulder stability

Steps:

1. Stand facing the wall with arms extended.

2. Squeeze your chest muscles, bringing your hands together.

3. Hold for 10-15 seconds, then release.

Remember:

- Keep your shoulders relaxed.

- Focus on the chest squeeze.–

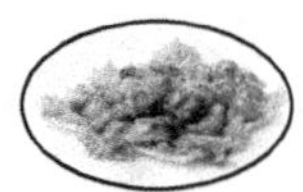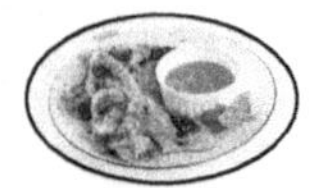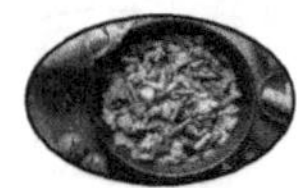

16. Wall Wrist Stretch

Benefits:

- Improves wrist flexibility and mobility

- Relieves tension in the wrists

Steps:

1. Face the wall with palms pressed against it.

2. Gently lean forward, stretching the wrists.

3. Hold for 15-20 seconds.

Remember:

- Control the intensity of the stretch.

- Listen to your body.

17. Wall Shoulder Stretch

Benefits:

- Relieves tension in the shoulders

- Improves shoulder flexibility–

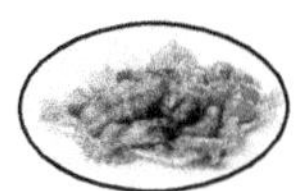 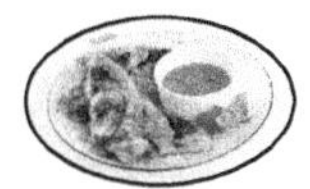 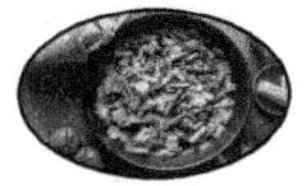

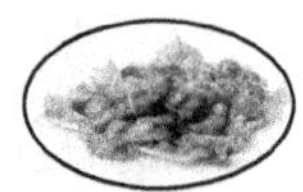 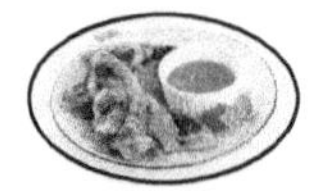 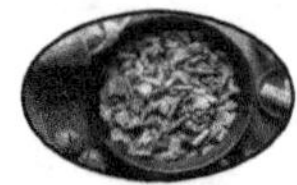

Steps:

1. Place one arm against the wall at shoulder height.

2. Rotate your body away from the wall, feeling the stretch.

3. Hold for 15-20 seconds on each side.

Remember:

- Keep your neck relaxed.

- Don't force the stretch.

18. Wall Seated Twist

Benefits:

- Stretches the spine and improves mobility

- Engages core muscles

Steps:

1. Sit against the wall with legs extended.

2. Twist your torso to one side, reaching towards the wall.

3. Hold for 15-20 seconds, then switch sides.

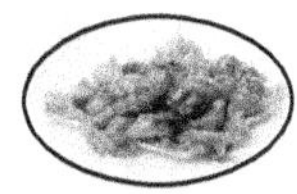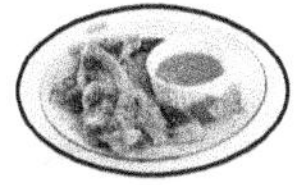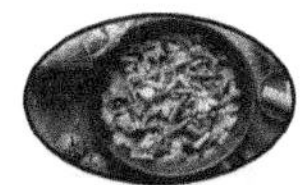

- Keep your back straight.

- Feel the stretch in your spine.

19. Wall Hamstring Stretch

Benefits:

- Targets hamstrings and improves flexibility

- Relieves tension in the lower back

Steps:

1. Lie on your back with one leg extended up the wall.

2. Flex your foot and reach towards your toes.

3. After ten to fifteen seconds of holding, swap legs.

Remember:

- Keep your back pressed into the floor.

- Feel the stretch in your hamstrings.–

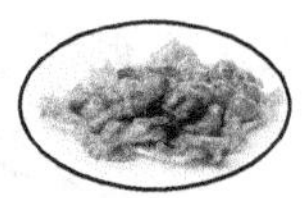 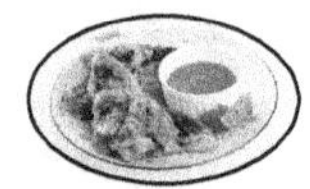 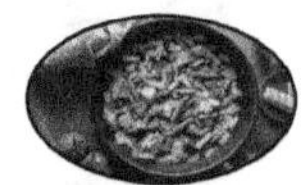

20. Wall Lunge Stretch

Benefits:

- Stretches hip flexors and quadriceps

- Improves hip flexibility

Steps:

1. Face the wall and place your hands on it for stability.

2. Return to a lunge stance by taking one step.

3. Hold for ten to fifteen seconds, then swap legs.

Recall: •

Maintain the alignment of your front knee with your ankle.

• Gradually sink into the stretch.

21. Balancing Bird Pose

Benefits:

- Enhances overall balance and concentration

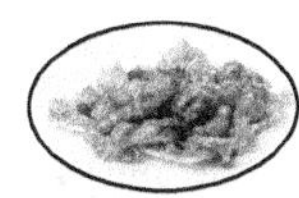 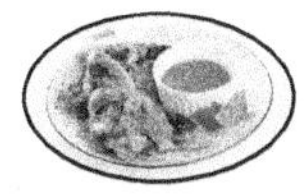 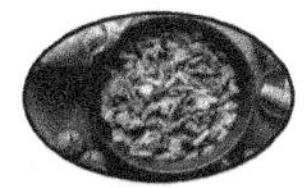

- Strengthens ankle and calf muscles

Steps:

1. Stand on one leg, lifting the other leg behind you.

2. Reach forward with your torso, extending arms parallel to the ground.

3. After 20 to 30 seconds of holding, swap legs.

Remember:

- Focus on a fixed point for better balance.

- Engage your core for stability.

22. Single Leg Deadlifts

Benefits:

- Targets hamstrings, glutes, and lower back

- Improves hip stability and flexibility–

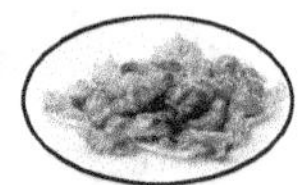 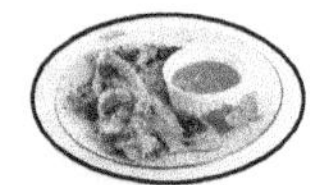 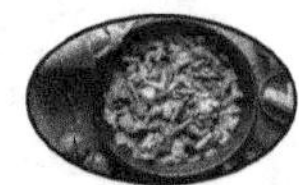

1. Stand on one leg, slightly bending the knee.

2. Hinge at the hips, lowering your torso towards the ground.

3. Extend the lifted leg straight behind you.

4. Go back to the beginning and repeat with the other leg.

Remember:

- Keep a straight line from head to lifted foot.

- Control the movement throughout.

23. Tree Pose

Benefits:

- Strengthens thighs, calves, and ankles

- Improves balance and focus

Steps:

1. Stand on one leg and bring the sole of the other foot to the inner thigh or calf.

2. Bring palms together in front of your chest.

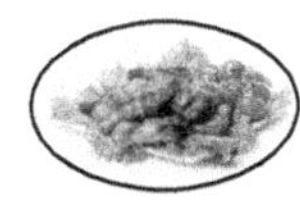 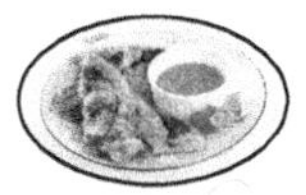 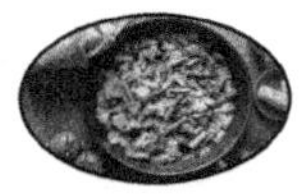

3. Switch legs after 20 to 30 seconds of holding.

Remember:

- Find a focal point for better balance.

- Keep the lifted foot above or below the knee.

24. Warrior III Pose

Benefits:

- Targets the entire back side of the body

- Improves balance and posture

Steps:

1. Stand on one leg, lifting the other leg straight behind you.

2. Reach arms forward, parallel to the ground.

3. Switch legs after 20 to 30 seconds of holding.

Remember:

- Keep your hips level.–

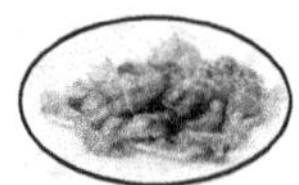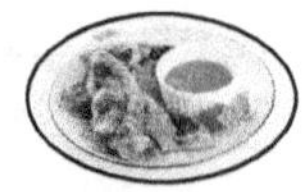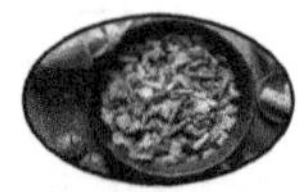

- Engage your core for stability.

25. Side Plank with Leg Lift

Benefits:

- Strengthens obliques, hips, and thighs

- Improves lateral stability

Steps:

1. Start in a side plank position.

2. Lift the top leg up and hold for 15-20 seconds.

3. Repeat on the other side.

Remember:

- Keep your body in a straight line.

- Engage your core for balance.

26. Standing Figure 4 Stretch

Benefits:

- Stretches hips and glutes

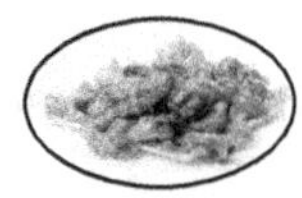 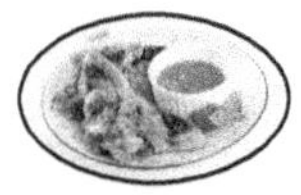 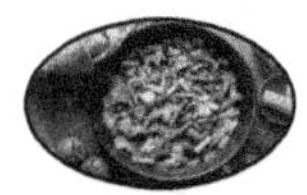

- Improves hip flexibility and mobility

Steps:

1. Place one ankle over the knee of the other.

2. Sit back into a slight squat, feeling the stretch.

3. Switch legs after 20 to 30 seconds of holding.

Remember:

- Keep your back straight.

- Control the depth of the squat.

27. Heel-to-Toe Walk

Benefits:

- Enhances overall balance and coordination

- Strengthens calf muscles and ankle stability–

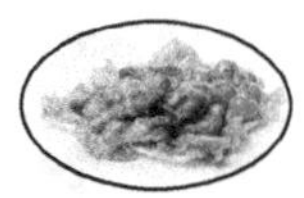 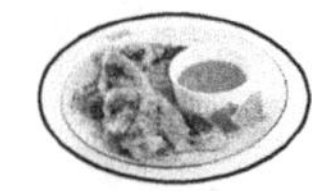 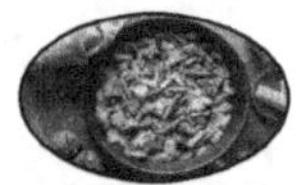

Steps:

1. Walk in a straight line, placing the heel of one foot directly in front of the toes of the other.

2. Keep a heel-to-toe pattern for 10-15 steps.

Remember:

- Focus on a fixed point for stability.

- Take slow and deliberate steps.

28. Balancing Ballerina

Benefits:

- Strengthens ankles, calves, and thighs

- Improves balance and posture

Steps:

1. Stand on one leg, lifting the other leg to the side.

2. Hold onto a sturdy surface if needed.

3. Extend the lifted leg in front and behind you, mimicking a ballerina's movement.

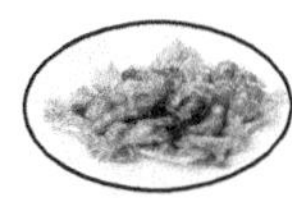 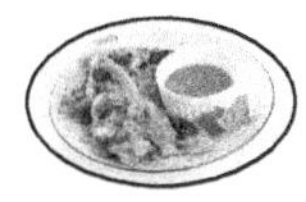 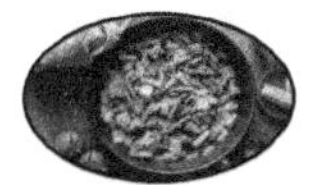

4. Repeat on the other leg.

Remember:

- Engage your core for stability.

- Control the leg movements.

29. Seated Leg Extension with Twist

Benefits:

- Engages core muscles and improves spinal flexibility

- Stretches the outer hip and thigh

Steps:

1. Sit on the floor with legs extended.

2. Raise a leg and place it across the other.

3. Twist towards the crossed leg.

4. Hold for 15-20 seconds, then switch sides.–

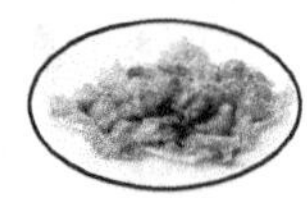 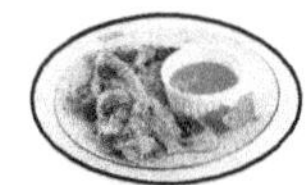 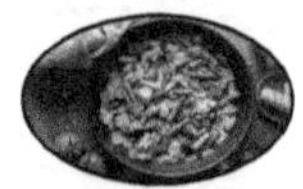

Remember:

- Sit up tall with a straight back.

- Feel the stretch in your spine and outer hip.

30. Standing Knee Hug

Benefits:

- Improves hip and knee flexibility

- Activates core muscles

Steps:

1. Stand on one leg.

2. Lift the opposite knee towards your chest.

3. Hug the knee with both hands.

4. Switch legs after 20 to 30 seconds of holding.

Remember:

- Stand tall with shoulders relaxed.–

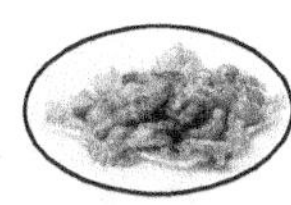 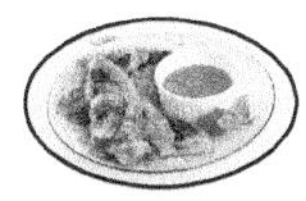 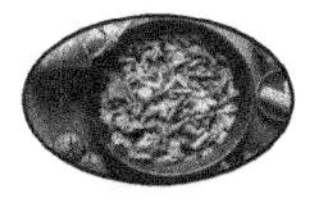

- Control the movement and breathing.

Congratulations on completing the ultimate 30-day balance challenge for women over 50! Incorporate these exercises into your routine for improved strength, posture, and flexibility.

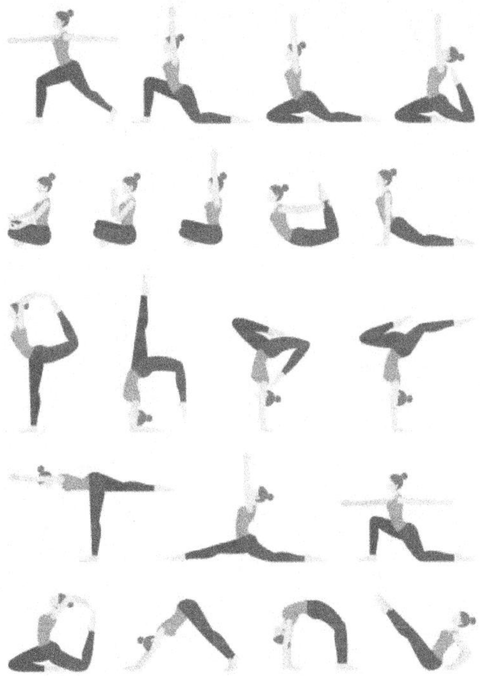

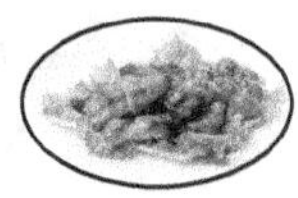 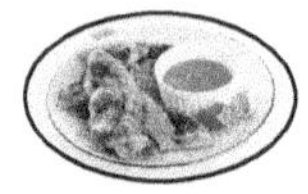 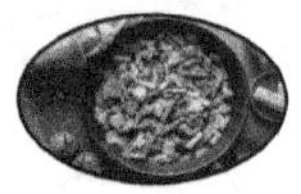

CONCLUSION

In the final moments of the 30-day challenge, as the sun dipped below the horizon in Harmony Springs, Amelia, Grace, and Olivia found themselves standing taller, stronger, and more balanced than they had in years. The echoes of laughter and shared triumphs reverberated through their shared space, a testament to the transformative power of commitment and resilience.

The benefits of this 30-day balance challenge extended far beyond the physical realm. As the women bid farewell to their daily exercises, they embraced a newfound sense of vitality that permeated every facet of their lives. The journey had not only sculpted their bodies but had also woven threads of empowerment, confidence, and camaraderie into the fabric of their existence.–

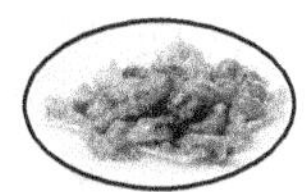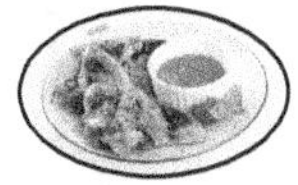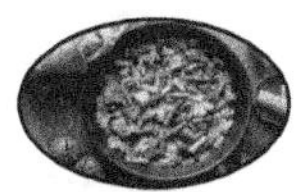

1. **Improved Strength:** The carefully curated exercises targeted various muscle groups, resulting in increased strength in the legs, core, arms, and back. This newfound strength translated into enhanced daily activities and a more robust physical foundation.

2. **Enhanced Posture:** The focus on balance and stability exercises worked wonders for posture. Amelia, Grace, and Olivia discovered that the subtle shifts in body alignment during the challenge had a profound impact on their posture, restoring a confident and upright stance.

3. **Increased Flexibility:** The diverse range of exercises incorporated into the challenge contributed to improved flexibility. Olivia, once burdened by stiffness, found a new sense of freedom in her movements, a flexibility that extended beyond the physical to a more adaptable mindset.–

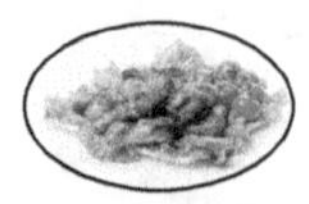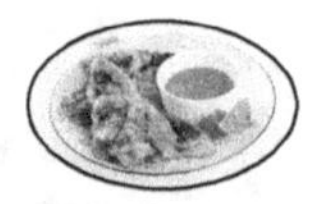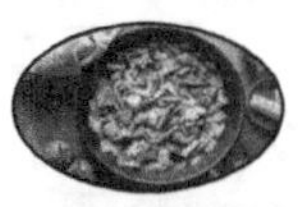

4. **Boosted Confidence:** As the women conquered each exercise, they experienced a surge in confidence. The ability to balance on one leg, execute challenging poses, and navigate the intricacies of the challenge instilled a newfound belief in their capabilities, transcending physical accomplishments to empower their overall sense of self.

5. **Revitalized Energy:** The rhythmic flow of movements and controlled exercises injected a surge of energy into their daily lives. The revitalization extended beyond the physical to a renewed enthusiasm for life's adventures, whether big or small.

6. **Strengthened Bonds:** The challenge was not a solitary endeavor but a shared experience among friends. The camaraderie that developed as they supported each other through the ups and downs of the challenge became an unexpected yet cherished benefit, fostering deeper connections.–

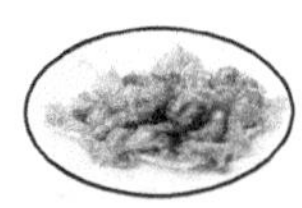 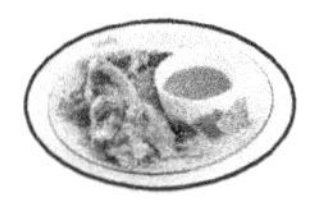 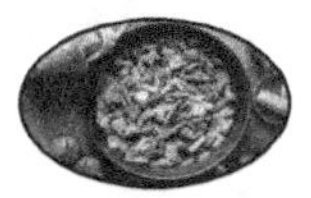

7. **Mind-Body Harmony:** The mind-body connection was a cornerstone of the challenge. As the women focused on balance and controlled movements, they found a harmonious synchronization between their physical and mental well-being, unlocking a sense of peace and mindfulness.

In the afterglow of the 30-day challenge, the ladies of Harmony Springs discovered that age was not a limitation but a canvas awaiting the brushstrokes of resilience. The benefits they reaped extended beyond the physical transformations, transcending into a holistic elevation of their well-being. As they embraced the lessons learned and carried the spirit of the challenge forward, the town of Harmony Springs became a living testament to the enduring power of balance, strength, and posture.

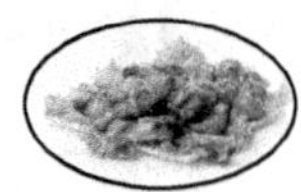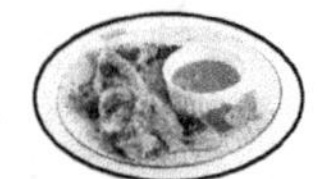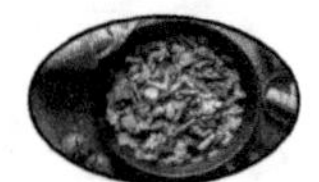

THAT'S WHY WE ARE SAYING THANK YOU...

"We know time is the unit of destiny, that's why we are saying thank you."

Dear Valued Customer,

we understand that time is a precious commodity, and we sincerely appreciate you choosing to spend a portion of it with us. Your decision to trust us with your purchase means the world to us, and we want to express our deepest gratitude.

Your support not only fuels our passion for delivering quality products but also contributes to the destiny of our business. Each customer is a vital part of our journey, and we are honored to have you

We strive to provide an exceptional shopping experience, and your satisfaction is our top priority. We would be happy to hear from you if you have any comments or recommendations. Your observations aid in our improvement.

As a small token of our appreciation, we kindly invite you to share your experience by leaving a 5-star review. Your feedback not only boosts our morale but also assists fellow shoppers in making informed decisions.

Once again, thank you for choosing to buy this book. We look forward to serving you again and being a part of your destiny in the world of quality and excellence

Warm regards,

JAMES CORDERO

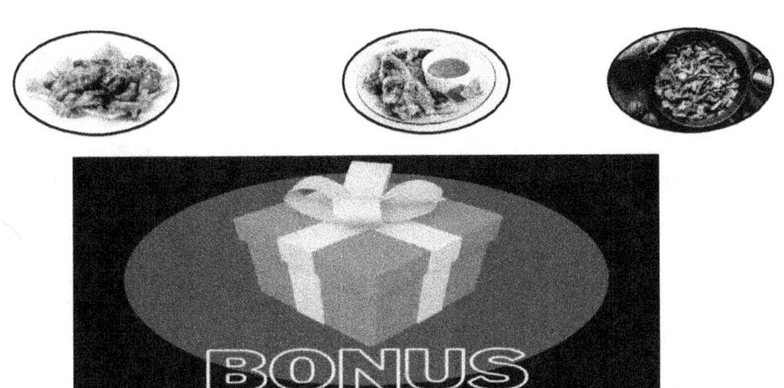

8 WEEKS EXERCISE JOURNAL

(paperback version)

BONUS 3; SUPPORT MAIL

Jamescordero@gmail.com

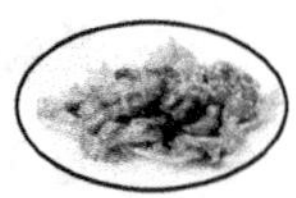 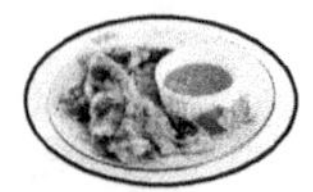 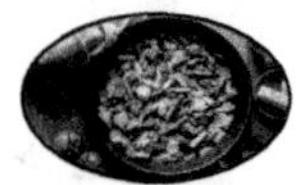

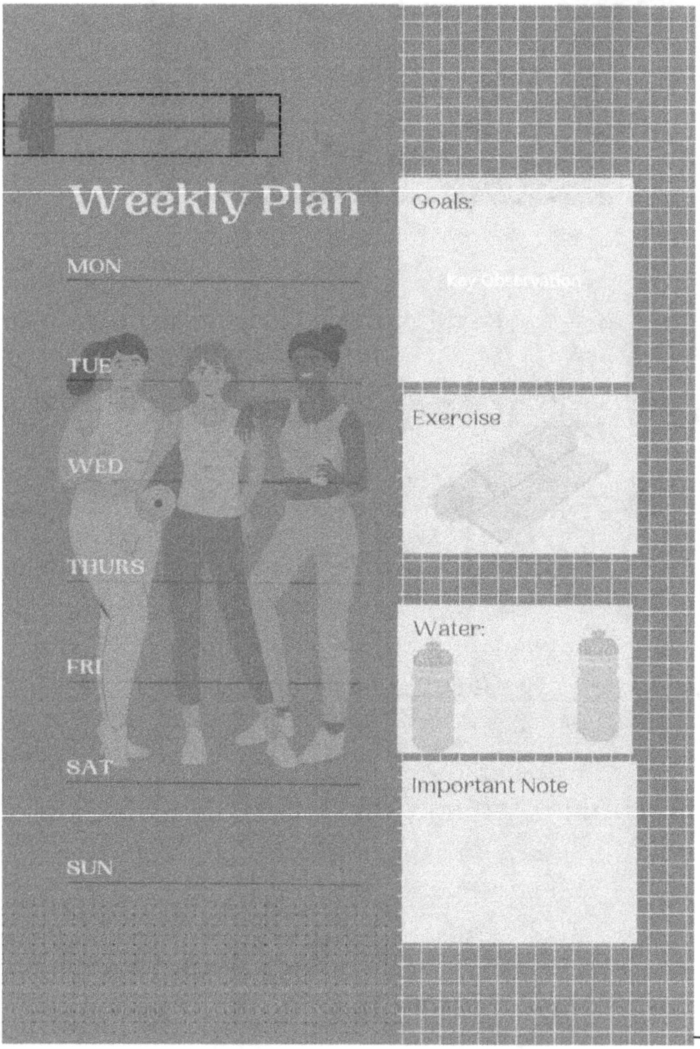

Weekly Plan

MON

TUE

WED

THURS

FRI

SAT

SUN

Goals:

Key Observation

Exercise

Water:

Important Note

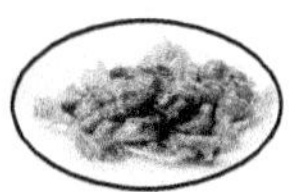 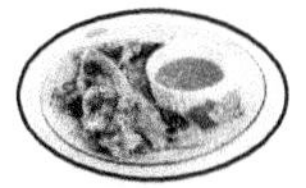 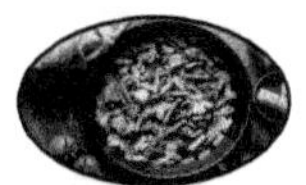

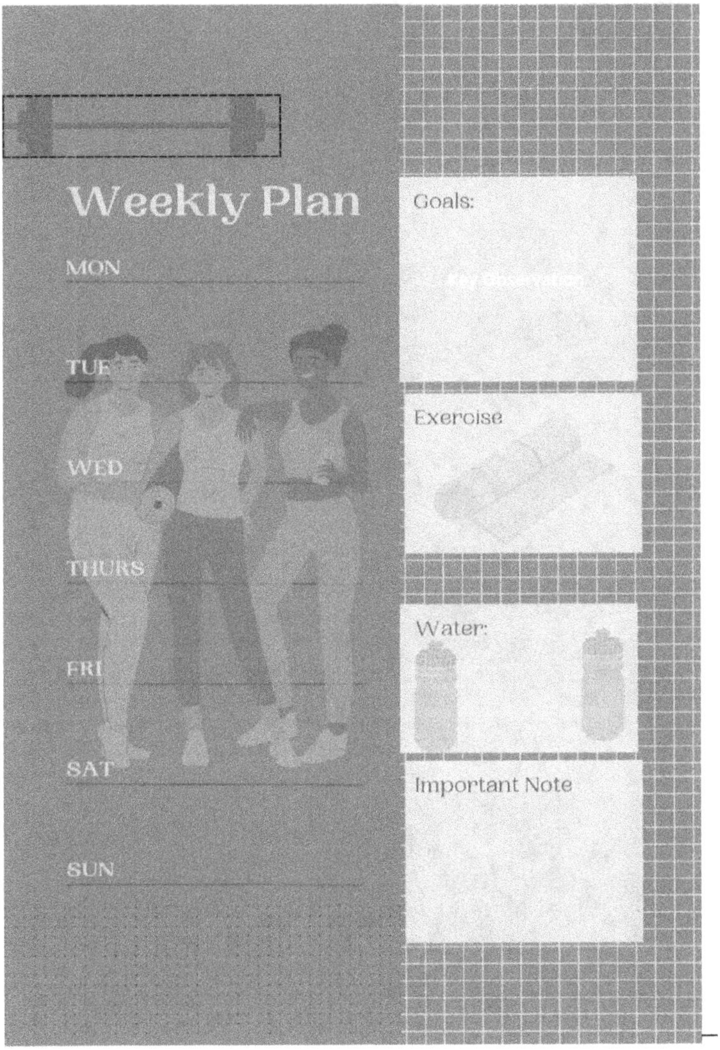

Weekly Plan

MON

TUE

WED

THURS

FRI

SAT

SUN

Goals:

Exercise

Water:

Important Note

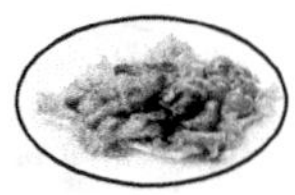

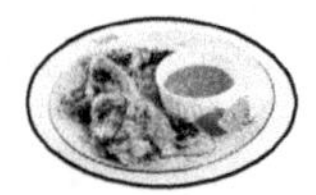

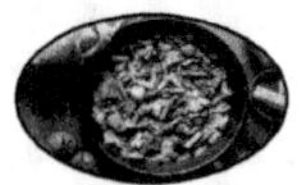

Weekly Plan

MON

TUE

WED

THURS

FRI

SAT

SUN

Goals:

Key Observation

Exercise

Water:

Important Note

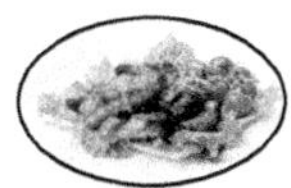 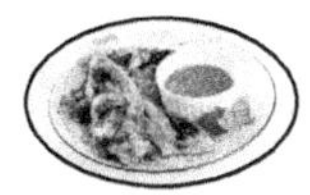 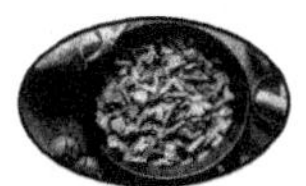

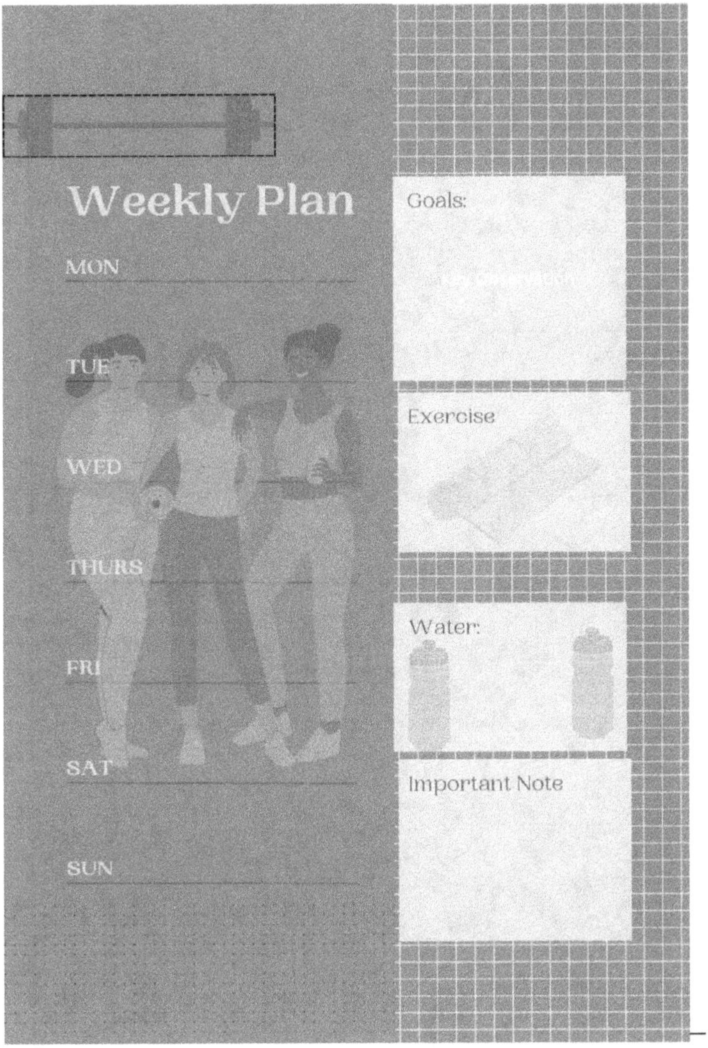

Weekly Plan

MON

TUE

WED

THURS

FRI

SAT

SUN

Goals:

Exercise

Water:

Important Note

Weekly Plan

MON

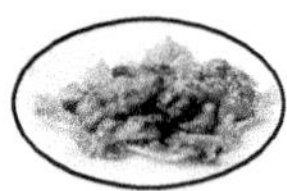

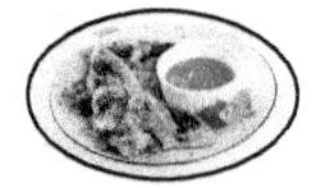

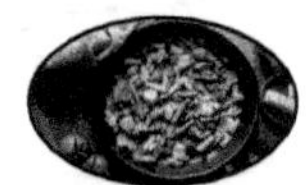

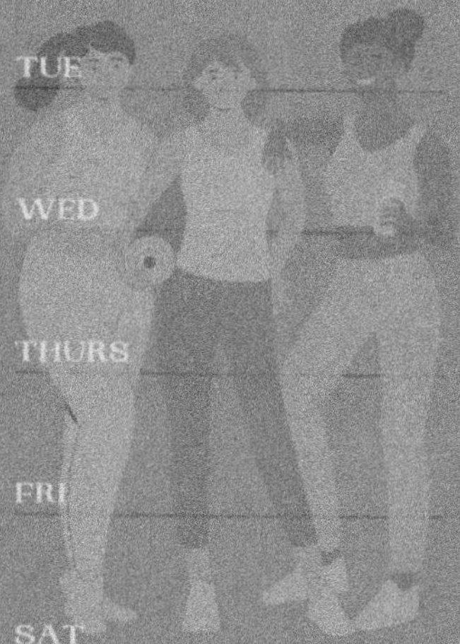

TUE

WED

THURS

FRI

SAT

SUN

Goals:

Key Observation

Exercise

Water:

Important Note

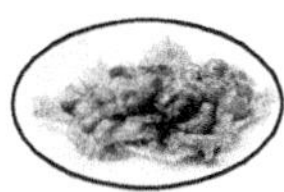 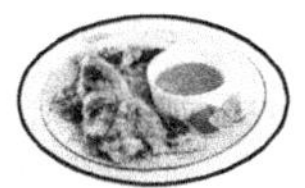 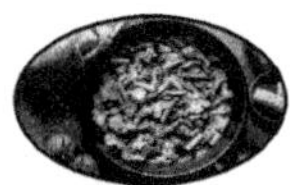

Weekly Plan

MON

TUE

WED

THURS

FRI

SAT

SUN

Goals:

Exercise

Water:

Important Note

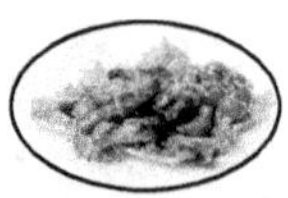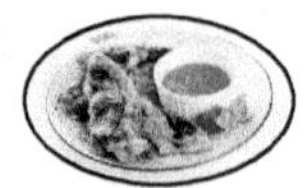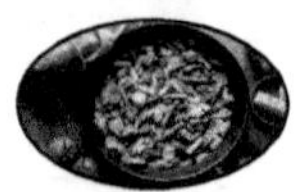

Weekly Plan

MON

TUE

WED

THURS

FRI

SAT

SUN

Goals:

Key Observation

Exercise

Water:

Important Note

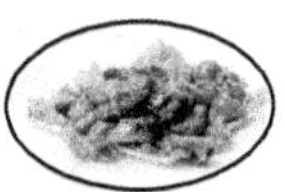 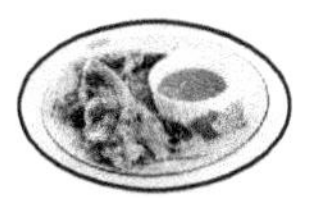 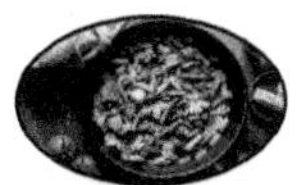

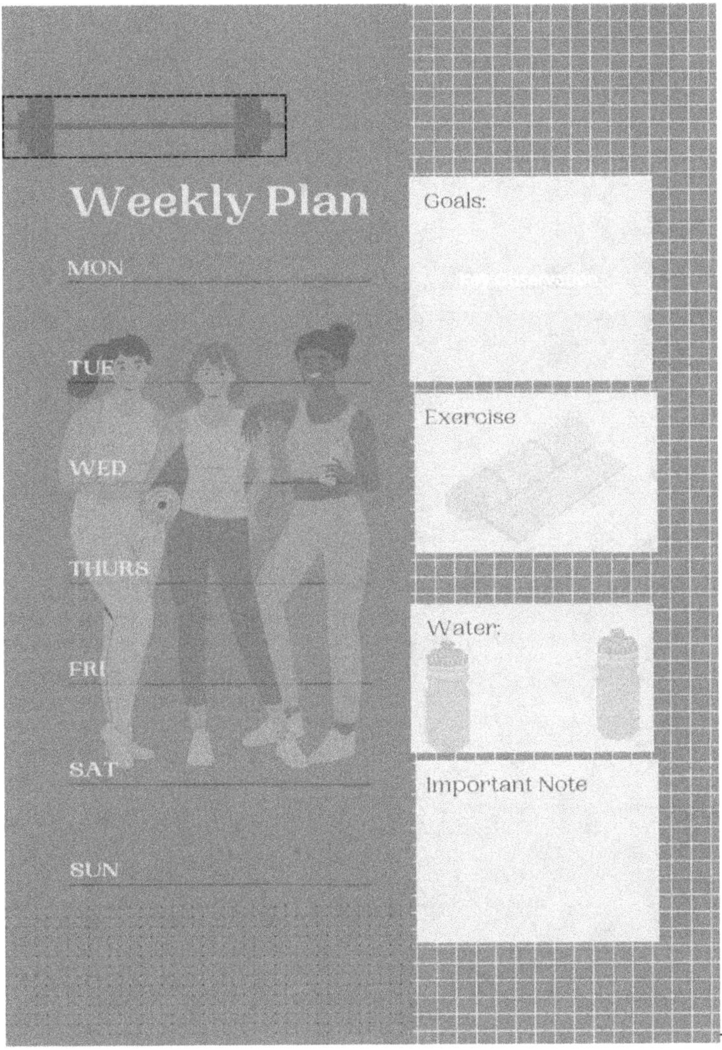

Weekly Plan

MON

TUE

WED

THURS

FRI

SAT

SUN

Goals:

Exercise

Water:

Important Note

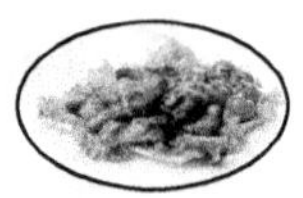 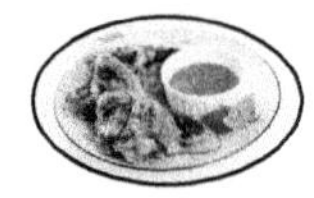 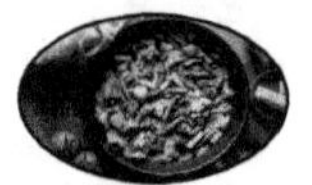

EXERCISE LOG

MONTH OF :

DATE	PRE-EXERCISE MEAL/SNACK	ENERGY LEVEL BEFORE		ACTIVITY/EXERCISE	TIME

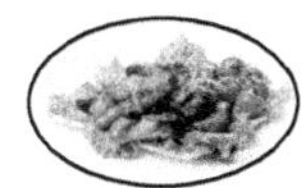 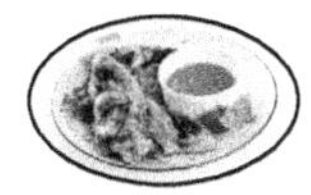 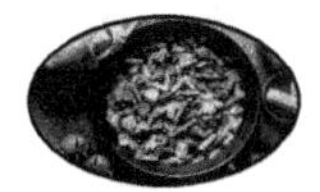

EXERCISE LOG

MONTH OF :

DATE	PRE-EXERCISE MEAL/SNACK	ENERGY LEVEL BEFORE		ACTIVITY/EXERCISE	TIME